I0787710

Regain your energy and your health in 6 weeks!

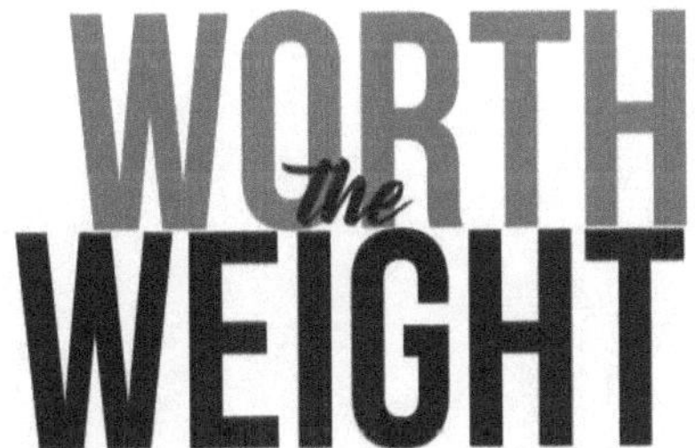

Kiesha R. Easley

This book contains advice and information relating to health care. It should be used to supplement rather than replace the advice of your doctor or another trained health professional. If you know or suspect that you have a health problem, it is recommended that you seek your physician's advice before starting any weight loss program. All efforts have been made to assure the accuracy of the information contained in this book at the date of publication. This author disclaims liability for any medical outcomes that may occur as a result of applying the methods suggested in this book.

ISBN-13: 978-1719364621
ISBN-10: 1719364621

CONTENTS

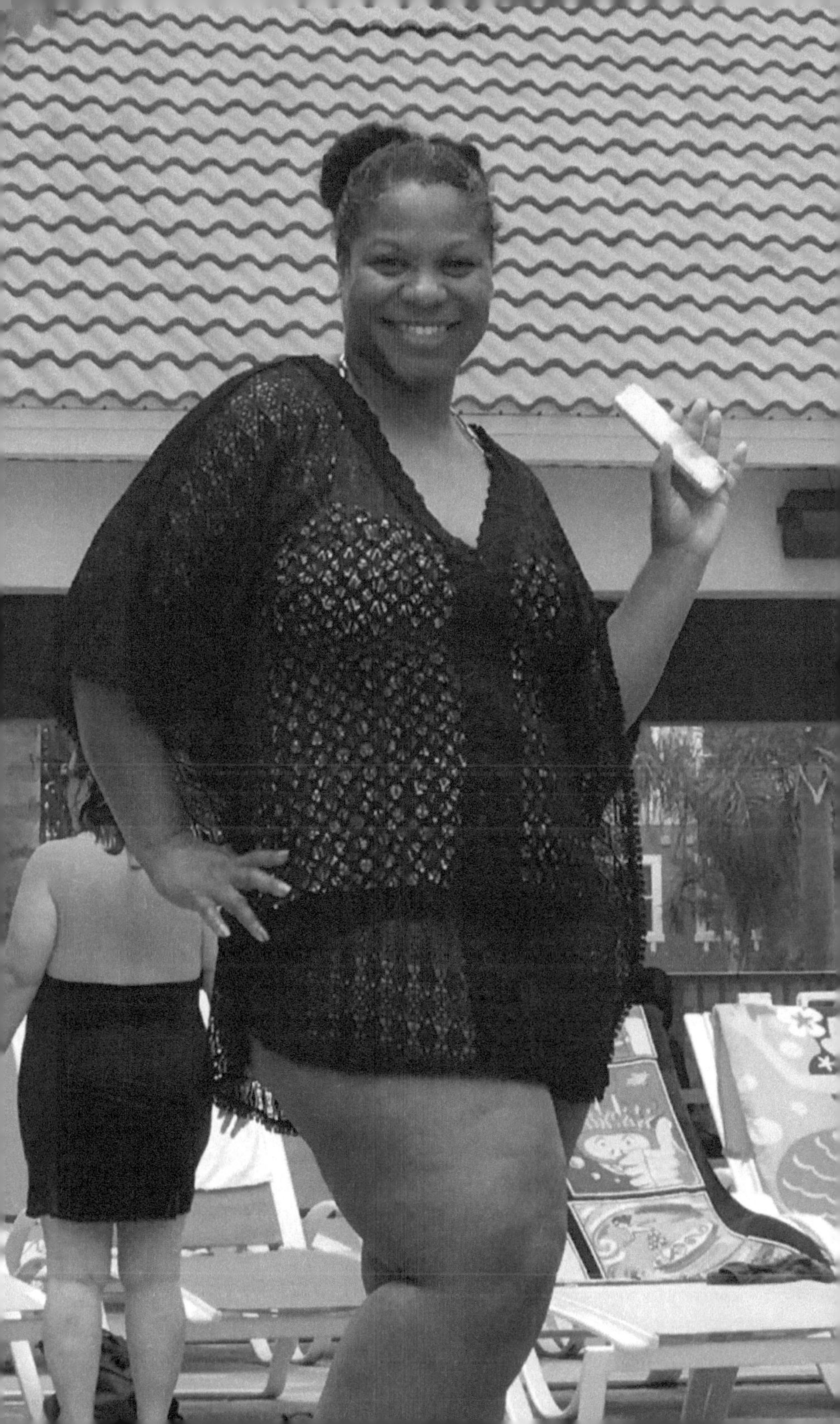

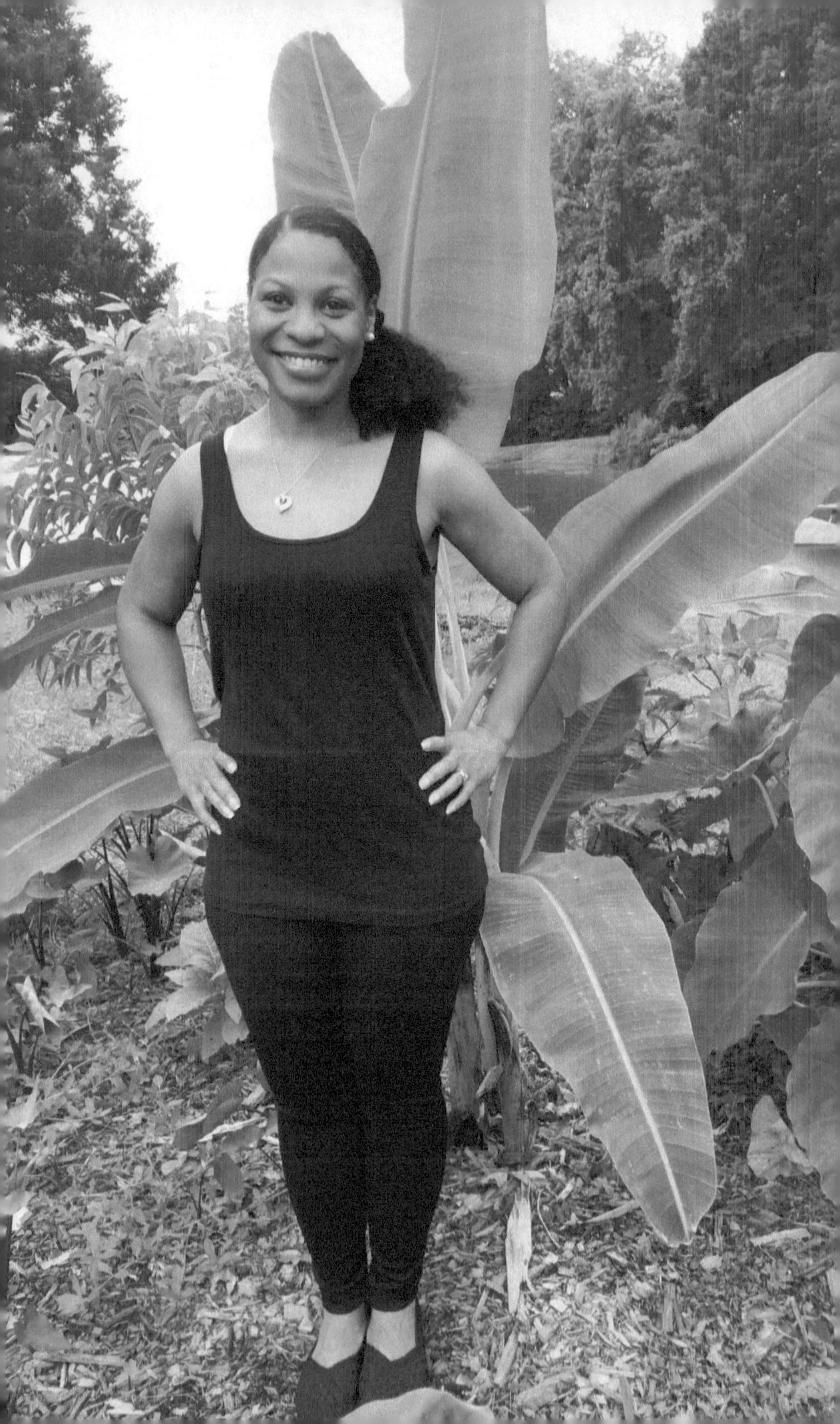

INTRODUCTION

Let me start by saying: *I'm not a doctor. I'm not a health care professional - at all.* I'm simply a regular person, who happens to be an English teacher, who got fed up with living in a constant state of exhaustion. My search for a solution led me to a book written by Dr. Steven Gundry, called *The Plant Paradox*. I thought I'd heard it all before, but it was as if this book woke me up. It revealed so much eye-opening information about food and its effects on health and energy levels. I'd been to doctors who couldn't explain my elevated white blood cell counts. I took tests that didn't reveal any real cause.

I tried increasing exercise and eating better, but nothing seemed to work.

After discovering that my eating habits and stress were most likely the source of my problem, I was convinced that if I could just follow the recommendations in that book, I would feel better. I wasn't so much concerned about weight loss as I was about feeling better.

So I finished the book and started the program. In just a few weeks, not only did I feel better, but I had much more energy. Before I knew it, I had lost a significant amount of weight and everyone started taking notice, so much so, that it inspired others to join in. First, my husband joined me in this new way of eating, then when my son and his wife took notice of how great we both looked, they joined in, too. They knew that if their middle-aged parents (who had been overweight for as long as they could remember) could do it, they could too. They changed their eating habits, started hiking and increasing their activity levels and now they both look amazing.

My results were so dramatic that people at work and church started asking me what I was doing. I've told so many people about Gundry's book and my experiences, that I finally got an epiphany - I needed to write about this so that I could share the story of my success with more people.

Even though I'm no health care professional, I have first-hand experience. I changed my eating habits in a way that made a huge difference, but is also sustainable. My goal, now, is to help others do the same.

My goal is to simplify the process for you. Throughout this book, I'll paraphrase some of Dr. Gundry's recommendations and link to valuable information he's already provided on his website.

I'll provide helpful strategies that helped me stick to the plan, but I still recommend reading *The Plant Paradox* yourself to get the full science behind the changes I made to my eating habits. Plus, you'll have access to all of the references Dr. Gundry used so that you can go and verify the facts, if you choose. (Disclosure: Yes, I'll get a commission if you use or click some of the links and make a purchase. If you prefer, don't click any links and simply search for it on your own.)

Get your doctor's approval, first
Of course, I must encourage you to see your doctor before you start this or any other program to get his or her approval.

If you take certain medications, they could be affected by changes to your eating habits, so you'll want to make sure your doctor is aware of what you're doing so that he or she can make adjustments accordingly.

Feel free to continue to read this book in the meantime, but before you take any actions mentioned here, get the okay from a healthcare professional.

CHAPTER 1
CHOICE + ACTION = CHANGE

In this book, I'm going to share the "Top 3 Actions" that helped me make my weight loss/health reclaiming journey successful. I wanted to lose weight, of course, but that wasn't the only goal. I just wanted to feel better. Sure, I didn't mind losing a few pounds, but my main concern was finding a solution to chronic fatigue and joint pain. I got tired of sounding like a drum machine every time I moved. Whenever I got up from sitting or lying down, my joints made a bunch of loud snapping and popping noises. I was worried that suffering from arthritis would be inevitable if I didn't make some changes. I knew getting healthy and losing some weight was a part the solution, but I kept dragging my feet. I just couldn't seem to get myself together.

As cliché as it may sound, I have made a weight loss resolution pretty much every year since I was about 20 years old. Even when I lost the courage to keep writing it down, it was always in the back of my mind. *This year I'm going to lose this weight.* Over and over again, same thing. I'd start the new year off trying to diet. I'd buy some new fitness gear. I'd read a book. I'd make an attempt for a few weeks. I'd overcome a few temptations to eat the wrong thing and go to bed hungry some nights.

When the time came to weigh in, I'd see some progress, initially. After about two weeks or so, maybe I'd lose five or ten pounds. I'd have a happy moment of victory. I knew that healthy weight loss happened slowly and I was okay with that. A few more weeks would pass and I'd weigh myself again. I'd excitedly hold my breath as I lifted one foot and then the other onto the scale.

In disbelief, I would step off and then on again, hoping somehow the number would change. After all of my days of struggling and starving, my weight had remained the same as before.

I'd think, maybe this is the "plateau" dieters experience. Then a few more weeks would pass and still, I'd lose nothing more, or maybe I even gained a pound or two. It was frustrating. Soon after, I'd stop struggling to eat bland food, get tired of starving and then one Nutty Bar at a time, I'd begin to give in to my cravings.

I'd shrug my shoulders and sigh; *I guess I'm just meant to be overweight.*

As I reflect on it all now, I'm realizing that I had accepted being overweight. I had a curvy figure and if I wore the right clothes, I thought I looked okay (mostly), although it was becoming increasingly more difficult to find the right pose for pictures. I found a solution for that, though - just stop taking pictures. That was an easy fix that made it easier for my weight to just keep inching into the 200s, 210s and 220s... I probably would have kept going if it weren't for the chronic fatigue, lower back and joint pain, and loss of ability to reach my feet comfortably. I worked as a professional nail technician in my early 20s, so I was used to doing my own pedicures, but for some reason, I would get out of breath while bending to attend to my own toes. My hip joints and leg muscles would pop and scream with pain as I tried to brush on a coat of polish. So, the time came for the next solution: I stopped doing my own pedicures and went to the salon.

When my joint and back pain got too bad, I'd take some pain medication. I thought I'd found a solution for just about everything except, I couldn't overcome the chronic fatigue. No matter how long I slept, I always felt like I needed more sleep. I yawned all day long. So, I went to the doctor. He suggested a sleep study. The sleep study revealed nothing abnormal. The blood work revealed no abnormalities. I kept trying to get more sleep. I even bought a new mattress, thinking that maybe it was to blame for my exhaustion, but that didn't work. I drank coffee. I tried doing less. I tried getting more exercise, but nothing had a lasting effect. It was the overwhelming fatigue that made me consider the fact that perhaps, this was a sign that I was unhealthy.   Something was definitely wrong, but nothing that could be diagnosed... yet. Left unchecked, I knew that the consequences could be diabetes, heart disease, high blood pressure, etc.

Last June, we took a vacation to Florida, our first major vacation in years. I bought a cover up for my bathing suit that I never took off - even in the water (see my "before" photo on the back cover). I was okay with that. What I wasn't okay with, was feeling so tired that all I wanted to do was sit down somewhere and vegetate while everyone else wanted to get out and see the sites and partake in the festivities around the resort. My family wanted to go out and find some excitement, rent the bicycles, go on an adventure, walk around, and go to the pool. I just wanted to take a nap.

My brain stayed foggy most of the day and I felt like I could fall asleep at will at any moment. I rarely felt good. My energy was always soooooo low.

The brain fog and constant drowsiness is what drove me to my search for a *real* solution. I was at a point where there was no other way around it. I had to figure out the cause of my fatigue. I had no treatable illness, so I knew my issue had to be diet related. I wasn't getting the right fuel into my body. The food I ate everyday tasted great, but it lacked nutrition. I wasn't looking forward to giving up sweets and snacks, but I was getting desperate. I was 40 and I knew that if I didn't get this health thing together soon, I might be headed for a future of suffering.

I felt a nagging sense that my eating habits were the cause of my problem. I loved the chocolatey-peanutty-crispy-delicious Nutty Bar, sure, *but was it worth shortening my lifespan?* It was my favorite childhood snack. I even had a special way to eat them - never whole. I gently separated them and enjoyed them wafer by finger-licking-wafer. As much as I loved them, the exchange of so-called "enjoyment" at the cost of my energy and health just wasn't adding up for me. I had to let them go. I had to make a choice.

My search led me to a video that explained how some foods that we consider healthy are contributing to our declining health. That video led me to the book that changed my life: _The Plant Paradox_. This is where I discovered easy to understand explanations of some of the issues I had been experiencing. It offered a practical solution: stop eating problematic foods (such as the Nutty Bar), stop taking medicines that do more harm than good, and start eating more nourishing (and delicious) vegetables.

I decided that it was time to change my eating habits for good. But no, I wasn't going on a diet; I was going to change my life by changing the fuel I put into my body.

Last year, I decided to start my wellness journey on a Monday. At my heaviest, I weighed around 230 pounds. By April 2018, I weighed 153 pounds, but most importantly, I have noticed an increase in my energy levels and have completely eliminated my lower back and joint pain.

I'm the only one who can truly appreciate the difference in energy and decreased pain levels. I could climb stairs again without feeling like my lungs were about to collapse. I could effortlessly walk faster and the best thing of all: I could paint my toes again!

Those were all welcomed changes that I noticed, but everyone who knows me has taken notice of how different I look as a result of my weight loss. In fact, that's one of the reasons I'm writing this now. Over and over, different people have stopped me to ask what I've done to lose the weight. They are amazed with my results and want to know the secret, because if I was able to do it after all these years of being overweight, surely they could, too!

That's what has caused me to reflect and think hard about what has worked for me so that I can share the same information with you. It boils down to the actions I took after I made the decision that I was going to change my health, but first, I had to make a choice: *keep doing the same thing and stay unhealthy? Or make some changes and improve my health?* I had to see it in those simple terms before I could truly accept the changes as something that I wasn't just going to do for two weeks, six weeks or even six months, but for the rest of my life.

The same has to happen for you. I can tell you about the following top three actions that helped me all day long until I'm blue the face. I can talk about all the benefits and give you all the little tweaks I made to my diet and how wonderful I feel as a result. None of it will matter. It will be nothing more than forgotten words, if you don't first make the choice to take the actions necessary to reclaim your health.

You don't have to accept poor health no matter how many diseases you've been told "run in your family." Don't let the past decide the future of your health. You can take control of the outcome right now. It doesn't matter how many times you have tried before – this time is different. This time you have a plan that will work if you choose to stay consistent and disciplined. This is the first time in my life of trying diet after diet that I've been able to surpass my goals. If you just do what I did, you'll experience the same results.

It's not about whether or not you can (have the ability), because you certainly can. The real question is not "can you?" It is "will you?" You must decide that you will do it. I won't give you a grammar lesson on the difference between "can't" and "won't" - you're fully capable of inferring the nuance. The point is that until you choose and then add action, you won't see any change. Choice + action = change. That's the equation that you should start working to resolve before you even read the next part. *What is your choice going to be?*

Your choices affect others

As I mentioned in the introduction, months after I started following this plan, my husband took notice of the positive changes in my appearance. Soon, he began changing his eating habits. He lost 60+ pounds.

His results were so dramatic that one day at work a co-worker who hadn't seen him in a while walked up to him and said, "I'm sorry for how I treated you last week."

Scratching his head, my husband asked, "What are you talking about?"

"Bill and I were chatting about you and when I told him that I thought you'd left months ago, he pointed you out to me! Last week when I came to help you, I thought you were a new hire!"

"Yeah, I do remember you were real short with me..."

"You've lost so much weight, I didn't recognize you! You gotta tell me, what are you doing?"

This is the most extreme reaction he'd received about his weight thus far, but it just goes to show how much of a transformation we have made.

Later, my oldest son and his wife took notice and wanted to know exactly what the two us of had been doing. I gave them the title of Gundry's book; they read it and have lost 20+ pounds that they have kept off. My son's cholesterol levels have returned to normal and he is now going on regular hikes and jogging around the neighborhood. This was something he struggled with because he's had asthma since he was a baby.

My youngest son, who's 12, had no choice but to eat the healthy food I was cooking and now he has more room in his clothes.

My mother in law followed the plan for six weeks and reduced the severe swelling in her feet.

The whole point of me telling you this is so that you realize, your choices aren't just about you. Your success could have a positive effect on your entire family. When people notice a difference in you, it influences them to make the same changes. So again, I ask: *What will you choose?*

If you're still reading, I'm assuming you've made your choice. Awesome! Congratulations! You've taken the first step. Read on to find out what to do next.

These are top three actions that had the biggest impact on my health and well-being:

- I stopped eating the wrong foods
- I reduced exposure to chemicals and medicines such as ibuprofen
- I started eating more healthy vegetables, meats, oils and supplements

If it's that simple, why are so many people still overweight?
I'm sure all of this seems like a no-brainer. It's so simple and straightforward, right? You might even be thinking *Duh! I already know all of that! Tell me something new! Tell me something I don't know. If it's that simple, I would have lost weight already!*

Chances are you already have an idea of what it means to stop eating the wrong foods. You've probably been trying to eat the right things, yet the scale won't budge and the health problems keep coming. If it were as simple as this, *why are so many people unhealthy? Is there something wrong with us? With our bodies? With our willpower? Why can't we put down the snacks and just eat right?*

It's because we've been misinformed!
For many years, I thought perhaps that I had a willpower problem. But I've discovered the real reason I was overweight and unhealthy was because I had been misinformed. I had been making good attempts to eat the right foods, but I was following the *wrong list.* I learned that some of the foods on my "healthy" list were foods that aren't really good for our bodies, especially in this day and age when we live more sedentary lives than our ancestors did. Some of the things I thought were "healthy" were slowly damaging my body and sapping all of my energy as a result. Some "healthy" foods were slowly damaging the lining of my stomach and sabotaging my immune system. Some foods such as sugar are addictive and cause cravings that are difficult to ignore and even cause withdrawal symptoms when you don't eat them. All of this made eating right almost impossible. You've probably been experiencing the same thing.

So, my goal is to help you get a better idea of what I've learned are "healthy" foods and which I've discovered are not. Some of the information I found was surprising and went against what I'd been hearing all my life, but I had a gut feeling (pun intended) that the new information I was learning was the missing link. It wasn't my lack of willpower, after all.

All of the attempts I had made to lose weight before had failed because of misinformation. If you've ever felt the same way, I'm giving you permission now: you can stop blaming your genetics or yourself for being unhealthy or overweight.

If you're ready to challenge your own ideas about what you believe healthy eating looks and tastes like, meet me in the next chapter.

In the following chapters, I'll explain the specifics of each change I made and provide some resources that will help you make the same changes.

CHAPTER 2
ACTION #1: STOP EATING THAT!

The most comprehensive list of foods you should stop eating can be found on pages 203-204 of *The Plant Paradox*. You can also find a printable copy of this at this link: https://gundrymd.com/plant-paradox-shopping-list/

Here's a quick list of foods to stop eating immediately. Read on to find out why they should be avoided.

DO NOT EAT List:
- Sugar or agave
- Wheat products (especially whole grain)

- Corn products (includes corn syrup)
- Brown and regular white rice
- Corn or wheat-fed dairy (and eggs), meat and seafood (don't panic, there are dairy products and meats you can eat)
- Potatoes
- Soy
- Goji berries
- Peanuts, cashews, sunflower seeds
- Squash family veggies (includes cucumbers, watermelon, cantaloupe, honeydew)
- Oils to avoid: Vegetable, corn, soy, grape seed, peanut, cottonseed, safflower, sunflower, canola, and partially hydrogenated oils
- Artificial sweeteners such as acesulfame K, aspartame, sucralose, saccharin, etc.
- Processed foods that contain any of these items

If you're like me, you probably would like to know why you shouldn't eat these foods. After, all some of them are foods that we've been told are healthy such as whole grain wheat, oats, wheatgrass, soy, etc. It may be difficult to give these up because of the so-called healthy association you may have with these, but it's extremely important that you avoid everything on the DO NOT EAT List.

Some of these foods contain lectins, which are toxic proteins that cause damage to the microbes and the lining of your digestive system. Your digestive system is the largest part of your immune system, so damage to it means that your ability to fight off infection is greatly diminished. It means that your body is in a constant weakened state, which sets you up for all kinds of disorders and diseases. So avoid the foods on the "DO NOT EAT" list as much as you possibly can.

Sugar and Agave

When I was young I remember my mother warning me that too many sweets weren't healthy. As a kid, I truly didn't care, I loved candy. For most of my adult life I ignored my mother's warning, I just couldn't accept the truth that something so delicious could be so bad for my health. It wasn't until I started feeling drained that I began to really take my mom's advice seriously.

Refined sugar must be avoided for two reasons:
- It makes our bodies store fat
- It supports cancer growth

Without going into all of the details, let me explain the basics: sugar causes insulin to be released into the bloodstream to break the sugar into pieces our bodies can use. When insulin is present, our bodies go to into fat storage mode instead of fat burning. This is what makes us fat.

The next downside to sugar, as uncovered by research mentioned in the "The Cancer Connection - and More" section found on page 256 of _The Plant Paradox_, is its ability to promote cancer growth. I'm not saying that sugar causes cancer, but cancer cells prefer it as a food source and are able to grow and spread faster when large amounts of sugar is present in the body.

So eliminating sugar from your diet is not just a good way to encourage the fat burning process, it is also a way to prevent and reduce cancer cell growth.

Wheat and wheat products
I knew that wheat products such as bread were fattening because of the starch content. Our bodies convert simple starches like this to sugar, so I knew I needed to limit breads and pastas. However, I thought whole grain was much healthier. It is not. According to Dr. Gundry, even if you don't have sensitivity to gluten, wheat, especially whole wheat is not good for our bodies. Whole wheat contains lectins that can't be removed through pressure cooking.

Of course, the lectins in wheat don't kill us immediately upon ingestion, but they do cause problems that disrupt our health and immune system. Wheat and wheat products cause inflammation and cause our body to attack itself. This is possibly the reason so many of us have autoimmune disorders. Adding insult to injury, wheat also causes weight gain. This is why it is the farmer's food of choice for livestock, because it fattens the animals quickly. That's what it does to us also. (Gundry 41-47)

The other foods on this "DO NOT EAT" list have similar negative effects and should simply be avoided, especially during the first six weeks. This includes avoiding meat from animals raised on these foods. No exceptions.

EAT WITH CAUTION
List of foods that must be pressure cooked:
- Tomatoes (remove peel and seeds)
- Peppers (remove peel and seeds)
- Beans, chickpeas and lentils
- Quinoa
- Basmati rice

If you must eat these foods, you should pressure cook them (with the exception of Basmati rice) to remove the lectins to protect the microbes and the lining of your digestive system from damage.

Eat in limited quantities (During the Lifetime Maintenance Phase only)
- Fruit (eat only in season and in moderation)
- Dairy (eat only "omega 3 eggs" or eggs from pastured chickens)
- Meat (eat only pastured chicken and grass-grass fed meats only)

Fruit
Limiting fruit may seem counterintuitive since all we've heard is how wonderful fruit is and how many benefits

fruit has. There are benefits to eating fruit such as polyphenols, antioxidants and vitamins and minerals. However, due to its sugar content - even though it is a natural sugar, it can still trigger an insulin response that could cause your body to store fat. Gundry suggests treating fruit as "candy". Yes, you can eat fruits from his approved list when you reach phase three, but keep this in mind: "eating fruit in season allowed our ancestors to fatten up for the winter." Fruit only recently has become available to us every day, but it was only meant to be consumed during summer to ensure our bodies stored enough fuel to survive the winter. If you start consuming fruit all the time, you'll kick your body back into a fat storage phase, so eat only the approved fruits with caution (Gundry 170-171).

Dairy Products

In the Lifetime Maintenance Phase, you can begin adding dairy back into your diet, but in limited quantities. You'll also want to try to find organic cheese and cream products from grass fed cows and preferably those raised in Europe, not in the US. Cows raised in the US typically eat corn - one of the most common genetically modified foods. Also, beef in the US comes from a breed of cow that produces a protein, called casein A-1, that can cause cancer:

> During digestion, casein A-1 is turned into a lectin-like protein called beta-casomorphin. This protein attaches to the pancreas's insulin-

producing cells, known as beta cells, which prompts an immune attack on the pancreas of people who consume milk from these cows or cheeses made from it" (Gundry 32).

European cow breeds produce A-2, a less harmful protein. Gundry also suggests using goat or sheep milk products, instead

Meat
The healthiest meat to consume is fish and other seafood. The next healthiest could be pastured chicken, duck or turkey. "Cattle, pigs, and sheep all carry Neu5Gc, which your immune system recognizes as foreign when you eat their meat." It can promote cancer growth, heart disease and autoimmune issues. So it's best to limit the consumption of meat from cows, pigs, and sheep. Even though meat is often the centerpiece of most of our meals, it's the part that presents the most risk to our health. For that reason, you should consider skipping meat a day or two every week, especially when you reach the maintenance phase (Gundry 157).

I typically only eat meat once a day at dinner time. On the days that I skip it altogether, I experience less bloating and gas and feel more energized.

Get your mind right
I highly recommend that you take some time to download the list from the website and thoroughly

review the list of foods to avoid. Then spend some time removing those foods from your home to make room for the new healthy foods you'll want to stock up on. You can't give in to temptation if you don't have any treats in the house. You can't eat what you don't have. So, take as much time as you need to get your mind right. Donate it, if you feel bad about throwing food away. Do what you need to do to separate yourself from food that wants to distract you from living a healthy lifestyle.

CHAPTER 3
ACTION #2: ELIMINATE THIS!

The next change I made on my journey to good health called for me to reduce and eliminate as many chemicals as I could from my diet and environment. I realize it's impossible to completely avoid all chemicals, so I'm not suggesting that you drive yourself crazy or become paranoid about every little thing. But your goal should be to drastically reduce your usage or completely eliminate as many chemicals as you reasonably can. That includes chemicals that you eat, breathe in, or put on your body. The greater effort you put into this, the greater the results will be and the better you will feel - there really is no way around this if you truly want to heal your body and regain your energy.

Of course, I realize that this becomes a very difficult task when you consider all of the toxins we are exposed to on a daily basis such as those found in our toothpaste, face wash, body wash, lotions, deodorants, makeup and other cosmetics. We are exposed to all of these just within the first few minutes of our day. This doesn't even account for the exhaust fumes and other pollution we breathe during our commute, the poor air quality in our homes or workplaces, or the drugs we take that we've been told are supposed to help us.

Chemicals you can control

Clearly, you can't get away from everything without moving into the mountains off grid, somewhere. All you can do is try can to control what you can. Limit as many of the following chemicals as you can. Your body will do the best job it can to handle the rest.

Try to eliminate as many of the following chemicals:
- **Antibiotics** - these should be completely avoided unless absolutely necessary.
- **Triclosan** - found in toothpastes, mouth wash, and hand soaps.
- **Pain medicines** such as aspirin and ibuprofen
- **Stomach acid blocking medicines**

For a full list of medicines and other disruptors to avoid, including an explanation of why you should avoid blue light, visit Gundry's website to read "7 Deadly Disruptors – 'Healthy' substances that actually harm you":
https://gundrymd.com/deadly-disruptors-plant-paradox/

Antibiotics kill the good bacteria you need to stay healthy. Avoid antibiotics, whenever possible. They don't just kill the bad bacteria; they wipe out the good microbes as well. It's difficult to recover your good microbes once they are gone and it becomes easier for the bad ones to take over. Also, try to avoid using antibacterial soaps. Ultimately, all these products do is make stronger bad bacteria that are becoming more and more resistant to antibiotics. This is very dangerous to everyone's health.

Pain medicines cause more pains in the long run.
Pain medications such as aspirin and ibuprofen are not our friends. The side effects of just one use are detrimental to the microbes and the lining of our guts. Have you ever wondered why they cause your stomach to ache if taken without food? That's your stomach's way of telling you something is wrong. The temporary relief in pain that these drugs may bring comes at a high cost. Of course, I understand that there are times when the stress of severe pain can be greater than the risk, so this is a decision you should make with a doctor. Of

course, I highly recommend that you conduct some research of your own, regarding the long term consequences of ibuprofen use so you can be fully informed.

If possible, you can try natural pain relief methods such as these suggested by Dr. Gundry: Boswellia or white willow bark. You should be able to find these natural remedies in stores such as Whole Foods or Earth Fare. They are also used in products called "Now D-Flame and MRM Joint Synergy" (Gundry 222)

Stomach acid blocking medicines
These medicines disrupt the natural processes in your gut. Instead, try Rolaids or Tums. You may have to take them more often, but they cause less damage. Dr. Gundry also recommends Marshmallow Root (Gundry 222).

Processed Foods
In addition to the chemicals mentioned above, it's also important that you avoid the plethora of unpronounceable chemicals found in processed foods. In addition to containing ingredients that the body wasn't designed to digest, processed foods also contain high fructose corn syrup, soy, wheat and many other foods from the "Just Say No List". With processed foods, you have no control over the ingredients they contain. So you might want to consider cooking your own versions.

Read all labels

Get in the habit of reviewing the ingredient list of everything you eat or use - yes, that includes soap and laundry detergent. Try to use less harmful alternatives and make the best effort to reduce or eliminate whenever possible.

Don't beat yourself up or put yourself in the poor house, but make the wisest choice you can whenever you can.

CHAPTER 4
ACTION #3: EAT MORE OF THIS!

The next major change I made involved making a deliberate effort to eat more healthy vegetables. As I reflect on my adult life, I could kick myself for neglecting to do this earlier. Aside from corn or potatoes (the worse choices), I rarely ate any veggies. I must have been out of my mind. I truly underestimated the power of food as it relates to healing. I just thought you eat to get energy and that was it. If you ate too much, you'd gain weight, too little and you'd lose weight.

I had never considered that the right foods could actually be better than medicine until I attended a conference in 2008. I met woman named Cynthia, a breast cancer survivor, who shared the story of how she cured herself with healing foods and juices. She wrote a book entitled, _My Seven-Day Makeover_ in which she shared her experience. She talked about feeling completely drained and frustrated by the treatment process her doctors recommended. She sensed that there had to be a better way, so she began conducting research to discover natural remedies and healing foods. She started eating those foods and within a week, she had recovered her strength.

So, I learned healing oneself was possible, but I just couldn't figure out how to practically apply the knowledge to my own life... until now.

Most of the foods on Gundry's approved list are healing superfoods. They have multiple benefits.

Younger Looking Skin
I have been told that I have a "baby face" more times than I can count. But, that tapered off once I hit the mid-thirties. I'm in my forties now, and all of sudden, now that I've improved my health, people are in disbelief about my age. When I tell them I have grown, married children and that my husband and I will be celebrating our silver anniversary this year, their jaws drop. When they finally accept that what I am saying is true, then they ask me for directions to my secret fountain of youth. I never get tired of hearing this or telling them

about how I was able to transform my health and apparently my looks, too!

Healthy hair, skin and nails + gray hair reversal!
Hair and nails grow stronger and faster when you are in optimal health. When your body is hydrated and healthy, you won't have to work as hard to keep your hair moisturized and your hair will have a natural sheen to it.

You don't have to believe this part if you don't want to, but it's true. I have discovered strands of my hair that are grey on the ends and black at the root. If I hadn't seen it with my own eyes, I wouldn't have believed it either. Last year, I had far more grey hair than I have now. The "before" picture on the back cover of this book was taken last June (2017). I just took the "after" picture in May 2018. I have not colored my grey, and I still have some grey hairs, but I definitely have less of it. I don't know all the science behind it, but I'm sure it has a lot to do getting more healing nutrients into my body while simultaneously reducing the strain caused by toxins.

Increased mental and physical energy and strength
I suffered from "brain fog" almost on a daily basis. I would walk across the room to do something and completely forget why I was there. Students would ask for something, I'd I completely forget just moments later. Now, I can honestly say, I have less of those

forgetful moments and I have greater mental energy and clarity. I don't feel like I'm walking in a haze, anymore, and if that were the only benefit, I'd probably be satisfied, but not only have I improved brain function, but I also have increased energy and strength, a stronger immune system, and have been able to maintain a healthy weight. You can enjoy the same benefits, too.

Stick to the "Approved" List
Here's a short sampling of approved foods that will help restore your health.

Vegetables:
- All kinds of lettuce
- Asparagus
- Avocados
- Beets
- Bok choy
- Cabbage family (broccoli, brussels sprouts, cauliflower, kale, mustard greens)
- Carrots
- Garlic
- Herbs
- Okra
- Olives
- Onions
- Spinach
- Swiss chard

Meat: You can have two 4-ounce portions a day

- Pastured poultry
- Wild caught fish
- Humanely raised pork
- Grass-fed beef
- Goat
- Lamb
- Venison

Nuts: 1/2 cup per day

- Almonds
- Brazil nuts
- Chestnuts
- Coconut
- Hazel nuts
- Hemp seeds
- Macadamia nuts
- Pecans
- Pine nuts
- Pistachios
- Walnuts

Oils:

- Avocado oil
- Coconut oil
- Cod liver oil
- Extra-virgin olive oil
- Sesame oil

Flours:
- Almond flour
- Coconut flour

You can find a more complete, printable list of foods you should eat and foods you should avoid at this link: https://gundrymd.com/plant-paradox-shopping-list/

Supplements

Our ancestors had a much more diverse source of foods, and so they probably were able to consume lots of beneficial vitamins and minerals that we don't have readily available today. So far that reason, Dr. Gundry suggests taking various supplements to fill in the gap. He offers lots of high quality supplements on his site, many that I have tried personally. However, even I sometimes get ovcrwhelmed by the sheer volume of supplements there are to choose from.

Over time, I narrowed down what I believe works best for me. I encourage you to conduct some research of your own to help you do the same.

Here's a starter list of vitamins and supplements that I take that I think you'll find helpful:

- Echinacea - immune support.
- Ginkgo Biloba - brain function support.
- Women's multi-vitamin - for overall health.
- Herbal Mood Support (Gundry product).

- Resveratrol - polyphenol that increases energy.
- <u>Primal Plants</u> (Gundry product) - vegetable blend, plus probiotics.
- <u>Vital Reds</u> (Gundry product) - polyphenol blend, plus probiotics that increases energy.
- <u>Prebiotic</u> - provides fiber/food for the probiotics (good microbes).

I believe these are the supplements that provide the best boost to my energy and brain function levels. But your goals may be different, so you should find supplements that help you achieve yours.

You don't have to use Gundry products, if you don't want to, however, I caution you to make sure you research the company to ensure you're not taking something that is going to do more harm to your body than good. The cheapest products aren't always the worse, but oftentimes, they aren't the best, either. So take that into account when making a decision about supplements. Some of the supplements Gundry recommends can be found on pages 273-285 of _Plant Paradox_.

Here's a list of some of the supplements he suggests with a brief explanation of each:

Vitamin D₃ 5000 - 10000 IUs
According to the <u>US National Library of Medicine</u> website, "Vitamin D helps your body absorb calcium,"

which supports bone health. So, you need Vitamin D to keep you strong, literally.

B Vitamins

There are multiple B vitamins that your body needs. "These vitamins help the process your body uses to get or make energy from the food you eat. They also help form red blood cells" (US Library of Medicine). These vitamins help you feel energized and vibrant.

Polyphenols

Polyphenols are important phytochemicals that keep your blood vessels healthy. Sources of polyphenols include berberine, cocoa powder, cinnamon, grape seed extract, green tea extract, mulberry, pomegranate, pine tree bark extract, and resveratrol, the polyphenol in red wine (Gundry 277).

Probiotics

The good microbes that live within your gut and assist with digestion and immune system function are called "probiotics".

Prebiotics

The compounds that the probiotics eat to grow and function properly, also known as fiber, are called "prebiotics". In other words, probiotics (microbes) need prebiotics (fiber) to survive.

Omega 3s

Omega 3 is a Fatty acid that is naturally found in fish and some plant sources. It supports brain and heart function. Aside from fish, other sources include flaxseeds and walnuts. (US National Library of Medicine).

CHAPTER 5
GETTING THROUGH THE PHASES

Now that you have an eating list to go by and an idea of things you should avoid, you're probably wondering what would be the best way to get started. Everyone is different so your process doesn't have to exactly follow my steps, you may make tweaks so long as you avoid the foods on the "DO NOT EAT" list and reduce exposure to chemicals.

Last year, I planned to start on Monday, July 10, 2017. I waited until I had finished the book and had a good understanding of the various phases of the program.

I spent the previous week preparing. I stocked up on ingredients I would need and ordered some approved oils and supplements. I got rid of food I knew I might be tempted to eat. If you're like me, and have a thing about wasting food, you can donate it or give away. I even planned in advance how I would handle eating during a trip out of town to my family reunion. I didn't want to leave anything to chance and end up hurting my progress.

I also reduced my sugar intake, not completely, but I avoided sweets such as cookies, candy, and other pastries. I did this to reduce the withdrawal symptoms. At this point, I was totally convinced that I needed to do this for my health, so there was no reason to do the "one last treat fest" that often accompanied my previous efforts. I realized that wasn't the best way to approach this new lifestyle.

3-Day Detox Phase

The first three days of the Plant Paradox program is considered the detox phase. This phase allows your body get rid of "bad microbes" and set the stage for the next phase of the plan.

What NOT to eat during the 3-Day Detox

- Dairy
- Grains
- Fruit

- Sugar
- Seeds
- Eggs
- Soy
- Tomatoes
- Roots
- Corn
- Soy
- Canola
- Fruit

What to eat during the 3-Day Detox

See pages 191-192 of *The Plant Paradox* for a more comprehensive list of foods to eat during this phase.

Vegetables:
- All kinds of lettuce
- Asparagus
- Avocados
- Beets
- Bok choy
- Cabbage family (broccoli, Brussels sprouts, cauliflower, kale, mustard greens)
- Carrots
- Garlic
- Herbs
- Okra
- Olives
- Onions

- Spinach
- Swiss chard

Meat: You can have two 4-ounce portions a day
- Pastured poultry
- Wild caught fish
- Humanely raised pork
- Grass-fed beef
- Goat
- Lamb
- Venison

Nuts: 1/2 cup per day
- Almonds
- Brazil nuts
- Chestnuts
- Coconut
- Hazel nuts
- Hemp seeds
- Macadamia nuts
- Pecans
- Pine nuts
- Pistachios
- Walnuts

Oils:
- Avocado oil
- Coconut oil
- Cod liver oil

- Extra-virgin olive oil
- Sesame oil

Flours:
- Almond flour
- Coconut flour

I followed Gundry's recommendations for aiding the cleansing process by taking Swiss Kriss the night before I started the plan. Gundry recommends Swiss Kriss, a natural laxative to help the body jump start the "bad microbes" removal process. It is a very gentle laxative when taken as directed. Without going into too many details, I'll just say that it has a very relieving affect and helped eliminate a great deal of bloating that I had been experiencing. It really helped kick things off nicely.

Challenges

The first three to four days are the most challenging. By the end of the first day, your body begins to feel the effects of the drop in blood sugar. You may feel extremely tired, like you could sleep or sit on the couch all day. You may experience headaches and dizziness. You may be tempted to take a painkiller, but avoid it at all costs. You may find that you are urinating more often as your body cleanses itself. You could feel hot and sweat more than usual as your body switches gears in the fuel it burns. For these reasons, it's best to start the plan when you have a few days off. I have summers off, so I was able to start on a Monday, but the best day for you might be on a Saturday or whenever you have at least two days off from work.

During the first few days, you may feel hungry. To combat those feelings, I stocked up on broccoli, which happens to be my favorite and salad. Every time I got hungry, I ate some steamed broccoli, tossed a salad, and drank green smoothies.

The recipe for the smooth, delicious, fresh tasting Paradox Smoothie can be found on page 330 of the text or you can find it at this link: https://gundrymd.com/plant-paradox-green-smoothie-recipe/

Before you begin, be sure to review the list of approved foods from Chapter 4. Pick up your favorite vegetables to snack on throughout the day. Eat as many vegetables as you want, but don't exceed the eight ounces of meat limit.

Stay hydrated!
You'll want to stay well hydrated at this time, so stock up on filtered water and herbal teas. I purchased a filter that fits over my faucet and a glass water bottle. I found one at Ross for about $6. You may use stevia to sweeten your tea during this phase, but try to keep it to a minimum. To relieve some of the tiredness, I took a daily dose Vital Reds as a supplement.

By the end of the first three days, I began to feel better. I could feel my body switching from burning sugar to fat. My energy increased noticeably and I felt ten times better than I had when I started. By the end of the week I began using ketone test strips to confirm that I had moved into the fat burning phase. Ketone test strips are used to test urine for ketones that are produced when your body begins to use its fat stores instead of glucose. This is a normal and health benefiting process that is not to be confused with what happens when a diabetic experiences ketoacidosis. (For more information, check out "What are Ketones?" at this link: https://www.perfectketo.com/what-are-ketones/)

It is not really necessary to measure your ketones, but I appreciated having some physical evidence that I was doing things right even when there were no noticeable changes in my weight. For this reason, you might want to purchase some for yourself. I've been able to find them for about $6 for 50 strips at Wal-Mart and for about $8 for 100 strips online.

Gundry recommends moving directly from the detox phase to Phase 2, so there are no gaps between the phases.

2-Week Repair Phase

Immediately after the 3-Day Detox phase, the 2-week repair phase starts. Two weeks is really the minimum, I continued on this phase for about six weeks. Even though *The Plant Paradox* only calls for two weeks, I really think you need at least three to truly get in the practice of eating right and establishing new fitness habits. During this time, you will continue to eat only foods on the approved list. The goal during this phase is to repair your gut from the damage caused by "bad microbes" and other toxins. According to Gundry, you could potentially stay in this phase indefinitely, but if you want to see even greater results and establish habits that will help you maintain your improved health and weight loss, you'll want to eventually transition to the next phase.

What NOT to eat during the 2-Week Repair

Grains

Fruit

Sugar

Seeds

Eggs

Soy

Tomatoes

Roots

Corn

Soy

Canola

Fruit

What to eat during the 2-Week Repair

See pages 201-203 of *The Plant Paradox* (or visit this link: https://gundrymd.com/plant-paradox-shopping-

list/) for a more comprehensive list of foods to eat during this phase.

Vegetables:
- All kinds of lettuce
- Asparagus
- Avocados
- Beets
- Bok choy
- Cabbage family (broccoli, Brussels sprouts, cauliflower, kale, mustard greens)
- Carrots
- Garlic
- Herbs
- Okra
- Olives
- Onions
- Spinach
- Swiss chard

Meat: You can have two 4-ounce portions a day
- Pastured poultry
- Wild caught fish
- Humanely raised pork
- Grass-fed beef
- Goat
- Lamb
- Venison

Nuts: 1/2 cup per day
* Almonds
* Brazil nuts
* Chestnuts
* Coconut
* Hazel nuts
* Hemp seeds
* Macadamia nuts
* Pecans
* Pine nuts
* Pistachios
* Walnuts

Oils:
* Avocado oil
* Coconut oil
* Cod liver oil
* Extra-virgin olive oil
* Sesame oil

Flours:
* Almond flour
* Coconut flour

Limited Dairy:
* organic ghee (clarified butter)
* organic heavy cream
* organic sour cream
* organic cream cheese

- eggs from pastured chickens

Limited Fruit (in season only): due to sugar content, you'll want to skip these entirely if you want to continue weight loss.

- Blueberries
- Strawberries
- Raspberries
- Blackberries
- Apples

During this phase, after about a week, you should begin to feel better and more energized. You could even notice some weight loss. Your hunger should decrease and cravings for unhealthy foods should disappear.

The first time I truly noticed the difference in how I was feeling was during the family reunion trip I mentioned earlier. After the picnic in Biloxi, I decided to follow my cousins to their home. It was roughly a three hour drive. Half-way into the drive, my cousins needed a rest, so we stopped at a gas station. While they stretched, I chugged my water.

When my cousin asked how I was managing to stay awake, I told him that the water seemed to help more than caffeine. As I thought about it more when we returned to the road, I realized, it wasn't just the water that had me feeling great. It wasn't an appropriate time to start talking about all of the changes I had made with my eating habits, but I knew that was it. I finished the drive and still had energy to spare. The amazing thing about it is that this was after a weekend in which I drove nine hours from South Carolina to Mississippi, dined with family on Friday night, went to the beach and attended our reunion banquet on Saturday, woke on Sunday at five in the morning to give myself enough time to get to the park and make some pre-picnic preparations. Then after a long day at the park, we returned to the road for this three hour drive to my cousin's house! And as exaggerated as this may sound: The next afternoon, I drove 14 hours to my hometown in Ohio to take my niece home and then 11 more hours back to South Carolina the next day. Yes, I definitely had far more energy than I realized!

In addition to repairing and re-energizing your body, this phase helps you transition to lifelong eating and fitness habits that will keep you feeling and looking great. Six weeks after starting the program I had lost over 25 pounds.

Swap out the bad choices for good ones
Since I adopted this new way of eating, I have been introduced to so many new delicious foods that I've been able to swap out all my old favorites for new ones. I really don't miss eating those unhealthy foods anymore, because I can quickly grab a satisfying substitute that will nourish my body rather than destroy it. Of course your favorites may be different

from my favorites, but you might find the following list helpful.

Foods I keep on hand
See recipes and instructions for how to use some of these ingredients in the "Recipes" section.

100% Unsweetened Chocolate (cacao)
100% Unsweetened Baking Powder
Almond Butter (No sugar or salt added, Non GMO)
Stevia Extract (with Erythritol)
Raw Honey (from my backyard hives)
Coconut Flour
Almond Flour
Wild Caught Yellowfin Tuna in Olive Oil
Sweet Potatoes
Sweet Potato Chips
Walnuts
Pecans
Almonds
Pistachios
Green Bananas
Frozen Blueberries
Salad Greens, including spinach and kale (sometimes from my own garden when in season)
Frozen or Fresh Broccoli/Cauliflower mix
Brussels sprouts
Cabbage or Cole Slaw mix
Avocados
Baking Powder

Spices
Pink Salt
Garlic
Onions
Organic Heavy Whipping Cream
Goat Cheese
Coconut Milk
Fresh eggs (from my backyard hens)
Fresh or Frozen Pork
Fresh or Frozen Chicken
Fresh or Frozen Wild Caught Whiting or Cod
Extra Virgin Olive Oil
Perilla Oil
Avocado Oil
Ghee (clarified butter)
Vanilla Extract
Mint Extract

My daily meal plan
Most of my meals are created from a combination of these ingredients.

Breakfast: Every morning I start my day off with a delicious blueberry muffin (made from coconut and almond flour) for breakfast. It's so filling that I rarely need a snack before lunchtime.

Sometimes, I eat salad for breakfast. Yes, I know, it's not what you would consider a breakfast food, but adding leafy greens to your first meal of the day is probably the best thing you can do for your body. Spinach or kale can be added to eggs along with onions to add nutritious flavor.

Lunch: I usually eat a salad of mixed greens with a vinaigrette dressing.

Dinner: I have a busy schedule, but I found it's super easy to create a healthy dinner by choosing one of the healthy meats. From there, I can add a salad (if I'm really strapped for time) or I can quickly steam some broccoli, cauliflower, cabbage or Brussels sprouts.

Snacks: When I need something crunchy, I munch on some sweet potato chips or I make my own fries from fresh sweet potatoes.

When I need something sweet, I melt some 100% unsweetened chocolate with some organic heavy cream, mint extract, add some stevia and whatever nuts I have on hand. I transfer the mix to small baking cups then refrigerate for about 20 minutes. See full ingredient list and directions in the "Recipes" section.

Lifetime Maintenance Phase

The Lifetime Maintenance Phase is the best place to be! It's where you will see the pounds (and your clothes) fall right off! This is what you will do to sustain your health and weight loss for the rest of your life. This is where you get to really celebrate your accomplishment and enjoy your new body!

It's also where you can begin to re-introduce some foods that may have caused you trouble before.

What to eat

I'm not going to provide a list here, because you still must continue eating foods on the "Yes List" and avoid most of those on the "No List".

There are two notable differences in this phase:
- Reduce meat intake to 2 ounces a day instead of 8 ounces.
- Slowly reintroduce some "Eat with Caution" foods

Slowly, means *really* slowly

Don't do this all once, but try reintroducing only one food for a week or two at time. One week you might try eating cucumbers again. If you feel okay after a week or two you might try adding tomatoes or peppers. *Do your best to avoid the skins and seeds.* Also, remember to pressure cook tomatoes, peppers, and especially beans before eating them when you're ready to add these back into your diet.

What to NOT to eat

Sorry, sugar, artificial sweeteners, potatoes and wheat products are still on the "No List." Continue to refer to the list of foods to avoid to ensure you don't cause yourself to backslide and reverse all of your progress.

Learn to read your body
It may take time, but during this phase, you'll begin to learn how to read your body so that you'll know what works for your body and what doesn't. I became more aware of how certain foods made me feel. If my energy was low or if I felt bloated, I'd take inventory of what I'd eaten in the last few days and almost always, I could name a culprit. Either I had eaten something I shouldn't have such as an overlooked ingredient in a dish or my body was fighting a cold or other infection.

Improving your health doesn't mean you'll never get sick, but you'll drastically reduce your chances when your immune system is running in top shape. I can honestly say, I don't get sick very often and I see getting sick as a signal that something is out of whack in my life. It causes me to take inventory of my sleeping and eating habits as well as my stress levels. I encourage you to develop this same practice. Anytime you don't feel right, take stock of everything you have been consuming over the last few days. Determine if you have been getting enough rest or if there's something causing you stress. Then develop a solution for how you will deal with whatever changes need to take place.

In addition to monitoring how you feel each day, you'll still want to monitor you weight or take measurements of your body. If you do this daily, when you notice a change in weight that's going in the wrong direction, you can take immediate action and get back on track quickly.

How to stay on track (and what to do if you get off track)

Periodically, you should try an intermittent fast or go as long as you can without eating, reduce caloric intake, or go a day or two without meat. Dr. Gundry suggests doing this once a week or every few weeks is a good way to help you maintain your weight loss and good health (232).

The benefit of intermittent fasting/meatless days

Fasting may sound counterintuitive or dangerous, but it's not. Fasting has been a part of just about every religion for a reason. It gives your gut a chance to rest and allows your body to reset. I am NOT condoning that you go on a starvation diet. This is not that. This is simply, deliberately setting aside a day to either avoid eating meat or a challenge to go as long as you can without eating breakfast. Try this at least once a month.

CHAPTER 6
OVERCOMING OBSTACLES

Losing weight can definitely be easier when you follow the plan outlined in this book, however, I can't promise you won't encounter any obstacles. In fact, it's best just to go ahead and accept that there will be rough patches and be prepared with strategies for dealing with the most common obstacles you may face.

Obstacles you may encounter along the way:
- Spiritual and emotional aspects
- Hunger and low energy
- Family and household challenges
- Financial challenges

- Time challenges
- Extra skin
- Recipes and meal ideas

Keep reading to learn how I dealt with each one. Feel free to skip to the sections that concern you the most.

The spiritual and emotional aspects

Embarking on a health journey is more than just changing eating habits. It's also about changing the way we use and think about food. The biggest obstacle you may face will be changing your mindset about food. Food is often the centerpiece of social functions and because of this many of us have developed strong associations of food with "good times". We all have a favorite food that our mother, grandmother or aunts used to cook when we were little. Now, that we are grown those foods have become a symbol of love and warm fuzzy feelings. It's even stronger if that person is no longer alive. Grandma's pecan pie becomes a way to remember and honor her during the holidays. Needless to say, these foods evoke strong feelings in us that we often don't understand.

In addition to evoking memories and strong feelings, food sometimes becomes a way to numb our emotions when our moods are low. Sometimes, food becomes entertainment when we are bored. There were many times when I ate when I wasn't even hungry, just to have something to do; to fill an empty void. I had to reflect on my eating habits whenever I felt an urge to eat something I wasn't supposed to. I had to be honest with myself and love myself enough to say: *No! I am not going to eat that because it won't solve the problem, but will instead create a bigger problem.*

I had to do some soul searching, and what I came to realize was that if I was eating to fill a void, I needed to get to the root of the problem. Filling our voids is something only God can do, but I was trying to fill my emptiness with food.   Voids are also a sign that we aren't working on our calling or that we've allowed some area of our life to get out of balance. *Was I eating because I wasn't fulfilling my purpose...? Or because I let the stresses of my job get the best of me...? Or because I was ignoring an issue I needed to address...? Something I needed to change...? Was I simply being too impatient...? Unrealistic...?*

As I spent some time evaluating my life, I realized that my job was robbing me of my joy. I thought about leaving the teaching profession altogether, but that didn't sit right with me. Teaching is ingrained into my personality, it's so much a part of who I am that I had no idea what else I would even want to do – aside from writing, nothing else sparks enough passion. So, I couldn't leave teaching, but I could change my environment. So I ended up switching districts. I didn't realize it at the time, but now that I look back, there was a lot of fear I had to face in order to make that decision.

There was no way around it, though. I had to face it and work through my emotions before my joy could begin to return. I'm happy to say that I am still teaching and enjoying it.

My road to healing was a spiritual one more so than it was a physical one. I couldn't have stayed disciplined on my own. I needed some supernatural help – especially since everywhere I seemed to turn, someone was offering me free sweets and pastries. The only way I was able to stay strong was by believing in and trusting in a higher power. God promises healing, and I had to believe that I could be healed– and this made all the difference. I encourage you to search your soul as well.

Sometimes, cravings were actually biological. If I wasn't eating enough vegetables; wasn't staying hydrated; yet was continuously flooding my body with chemicals and junk food, of course my body was going to send out a signal to eat. My body did this in hopes that I was actually going eat something nourishing, but when that didn't happen, the signals kept coming.

Those issues were resolved when I finally started nourishing my body. This is 80% of the battle. If you can nourish your body, you will have greater spiritual strength when temptation comes. You'll have the strength to think about why you feel the need to eat when you're not hungry. You'll have the strength to take control, rather than let your cravings control you.

For the other 20% of emotionally driven cravings, I recommend taking some time to take care of yourself and get your life back in balance. I found that when I worked myself too hard without allowing myself times of rest and recreation, my mood would bottom out quickly and I'd find myself turning to food to boost my mood. That's not a healthy way to live life and it's not the way God intended for us to live.

Food is NOT entertainment and food is NOT a mood enhancer.
We have to find new ways to relax and do what we really love instead of stuffing our faces. I had to reconnect with my art hobby. Painting soothes me far better and longer than a Nutty Bar ever could! I also love to dance and the beautiful thing about it is that it helped me exercise without feeling like I was exercising – so it had multiple benefits that eating junk food never had.

So, I encourage you to reconnect or spend some time finding an entertaining and relaxing activity that you love.

Of course, there will be times when food will be part of a celebration and of course, you should enjoy, but be honest with yourself about what you're eating and adhere to reasonable limits. During the Thanksgiving and Christmas holidays I enjoyed pieces of my favorite cakes and pies, but when the season was over, I went right back to disciplined eating habits. I had to get back on track – I couldn't let all of my progress and hard work go to waste. Also, it wasn't without a lesson: I tried to eat some oatmeal cookies and got sick as a dog. This was a wakeup call and reminder to avoid oats completely.

I encourage you to do some soul searching and thinking about how much food controls your day and your actions. Are you elevating food to a status that it shouldn't be in? Are you positioning food as the center of your life? Has the taste become more important than your well-being?

Make a plan for how you will deal with the emotional cravings that may come along. It might be time to find a hobby or rearrange some things in your life. After all, you can't expect to have a healthy body if you aren't living a healthy life.

If you have toxic relationships or habits, you'll need to treat them like the foods on the "NO List" – get rid of them. If you're struggling to do this, you'll need to go back to the first chapter and make a decision. I encourage you to choose to be healthy.

You really can't make any major changes or accomplish much in life, if you don't feel well. Get your mind right, eat right and your body will follow.

Hunger and Low Energy

Since eating is not a one-time deal, it is inevitable at some point that you will become hungry. The problem comes when it happens at a time when you're not adequately prepared. If you let yourself get to a point when you're too hungry to think, you might ultimately eat something you shouldn't and throw your body off course. To avoid this, you need a plan for how you will handle those times when you'll find yourself needing to eat when there are no healthy options around.

Stay on top of hunger.
Carry healthy snacks everywhere you go. I understand that steamed veggies and baked fish aren't portable items that are easy to eat anytime. So, it's a good idea to keep bags of approved nuts, raw veggies such as broccoli or cauliflower with you at all times.

I keep a spare bag of walnuts in my purse and book bag. That way, when I find myself needing some energy, I don't have to expend any energy looking for healthy options.

Avoid dehydration
Since thirst can trick you into thinking you're hungry, it's best to not let yourself get dehydrated. Dehydration

is the biggest reason why many of us feel tired. It's also the most ignored problem. We tend not to realize how serious dehydration can be. When your body, which is 85% water by the way, can't get enough water, it can't circulate your blood properly. That means your cells aren't getting fed the nutrients that the blood carries as efficiently as they should.

When your body goes too long this way, it weakens the system, leaving you more susceptible to the effects of stress and toxins that come with day to day living. Prolonged dehydration doesn't just leave you feeling drained of your precious energy, it can make you sick.

Even worse, dehydration can increase your risk of heart attack. According to the American Heart Association website, "This condition causes blood vessels to narrow and blood to thicken, raising risk for blood clots." Imagine dying from a heart attack caused by dehydration, a highly preventable condition. It's just not worth it. (http://www.heart.org)

I realize most people don't even drink plain water on a regular basis. I understand water can seem boring compared to all of the delicious beverages there are to choose from. But truly, it's the perfect beverage for your body. The more you make yourself drink water instead, the more you'll get used to only drinking water. Coffee and tea are still healthy beverages, but they shouldn't be a substitute.

Here are some strategies that can help increase your water intake:

Find a cute glass water bottle

Glass bottles are BPA free and don't add that "plastic taste" to your water. Plus, it naturally keeps it cool longer. I like the water bottles that have the silicone wraps that protect it from breaking so easily if dropped. I encourage you to find a cute one in your favorite color (I love pink!).

Add lemon, lime or mint

Sometimes you just need a little flavor to help you out. These are the best choices because they don't add any sugar. They also add vitamin C and other nutrients that are beneficial to your body.

Challenge yourself!

Challenge yourself to drink at least 24 ounces of water before drinking any other flavored beverages. Of course, make sure those beverages don't contain any sugar or artificial sweeteners. Instead, use stevia or a little honey.

I know it can be hard to make yourself drink enough water, but it's worth it. At first, you may have to make yourself drink more and it may seem as if you're forcing yourself, but after a few days to a week to drinking more water, you'll begin to crave just pure water.

Family & Household Challenges

Adhering to a new eating plan is already difficult enough, but it can be even more challenging if you have family members in your household who don't want to join your new way of eating. I realize it may be difficult serving two different meals, but you shouldn't try to force any adult to do something they don't want to. Now, other hand, you could gently transition your children into eating healthily.

It's best to plan ahead and develop solutions for how you will handle these challenges before they occur.

Here are some tips that may help:

Prepare healthy options along with your family's regular meal. You'll still be able to eat the healthy "Gundry approved" items while satisfying your family's needs.

Plan how you will handle the temptation in advance. It's important that you go ahead and accept that temptation will come. Yes, you'll want to create as much of a safe haven in your home as possible, but there may be times when you'll have to watch your friends or the members in your household eat pizza while you're eating a salad. Develop a mental strategy that will help you cope. Whenever possible, make sure you eat ahead of time so that you're not hungry. If that's not possible, keep some nuts with you (pecans, pistachios, walnut, etc.) and munch on them to keep you from caving.

Plan how you will handle feeling awkward during social gatherings or other social events where food will be involved. Not eating certain foods or not eating at all during a gathering where food is served can leave you feeling a bit awkward, so you need to be prepared for how you will handle your own feelings and also how you might address questions other people may ask. You don't want to let your awkwardness cause you to cave and eat something you shouldn't so you plan your response ahead of time. If someone asks why you're not eating what's being served, you could tell them that you have diet restrictions that won't allow certain foods. If it's a family gathering you could discreetly eat the approved items only. The more you practice this, the more at ease you will become.

Financial Challenges

We all know that it's cheaper to buy cookies, chips, and hamburgers than it is to buy a fresh salad. I had to accept this for myself: Healthy food is more expensive because it is "actually" food - everything else is pretty much just a bunch of food-flavored chemicals.

A salad costs more because lots of hands are involved in growing, nurturing, harvesting, packing, delivering and maintaining its freshness. Real food goes bad quickly because even bacteria can recognize healthy food. Have you ever wondered why some snacks never go bad? It means that microbes have rejected it as a food source, and we should too!

I understand, however, that knowing and accepting all of this doesn't change the balance of your bank account or your budget.

I understand the struggle, so here are strategies I used to fund my new eating habits:

Grow or raise your own food
You may or may not have noticed that in my list of foods I keep on hand were some items that I grow or raise myself. Initially, this may not seem practical, however, if think it about, it's a must. Here's why: growing your own food allows you to eliminate pesticides and herbicides. It allows you benefit from the natural and healthy microbes that can only come from your local soil, and you decide what to feed your livestock. That means you can eliminate GMO products such as corn and soy from their feed. In other words, it's an investment that is not just beneficial financially, but is one of the healthiest choices you can make.

Let me also add, that when you grow your own food means you'll get to eat high quality and some of the most delicious food you'll ever taste. I thought I hated Brussels sprouts, until I grew my own and got a chance to taste them at the peak of their freshness and in the most nutrient dense state. Everything tastes better when it comes fresh from your own backyard, I promise, you'll become so spoiled by this that you'll never want to eat any other way.

So when the season permits, I'm always growing kale and salad greens. I grow my own ginger, rosemary, mint, sweet potatoes, blackberries, blueberries, mulberries, strawberries, apples, citrus, peaches, nectarines, pears, plums, and banana. In the past, I've grown onions, garlic and asparagus, a wonderful perennial that grows back every year, with little maintenance.

We also raise our own chickens for their eggs and honeybees for raw honey. I've never tasted eggs so rich and flavorful before - they barely require any seasoning. Every batch of honey we harvest has its own unique flavor that is unlike anything you've ever tasted. Once you taste raw honey from your own backyard, you'll wonder how you ever tolerated the stuff that comes out of those bears in the grocery store. There's no comparison!

So challenge yourself to add this strategy to help you save money and gain so many other benefits in the process. If you need some tips for how to start a garden, you can visit our website:
http://easilygrowngarden.com/category/gardening-tips/

Or feel free to conduct a search online or YouTube, there's tons of information out there.

Make your own

Next to growing your own food, making your own is also a great way to save tons of money. It's also the best way to ensure there are no extra chemicals or ingredients that you shouldn't be eating. It may take a little bit more time, but with the right planning and storage methods, you can make your own delicious food that will help you stay healthy.

I've included a few of my adaptations of recipes in the "Recipes" section of this book, but I encourage you to adapt your own recipes by swapping out the unhealthy foods for healthy substitutes. For example, instead of making muffins with wheat flour, you can swap out the wheat flour for coconut and almond flour (You can find the full recipe in the "Recipes" section).

Don't be afraid to play around with ingredients and challenge your ideas of which foods you can mix together. My son wanted chili cheese fries, but white potatoes are off limits, so I used sweet potatoes to make my own fries, ground turkey and a combination of seasonings to make the chili. I added organic sour cream and cheddar cheese and made a healthy alternative that he thoroughly enjoyed.

All you need is a little creativity and willingness to experiment.

Here's a list of items you should consider making for yourself.
- Chocolate candy
- Ghee (clarified butter)
- Ice Cream
- Salad Dressing
- Sweet potato fries
- Whipped Cream

These are just a few suggestions. Consider your preferences and conduct some research, if needed, to find recipes that you can tweak to remove unhealthy ingredients.

Buy only what you need for the week
Yes, healthy food costs more, but you'll need less because it nourishes more. It's easy to "stock up" on all those unhealthy foods because they are cheaper and they never go bad - so in many ways you can spend more than you planned on junk. On the other hand, fresh food doesn't store well - salads greens won't last more than a week in the fridge, so you actually spend less when you buy on an "as needed basis."

Stock up on frozen goods when you find sales.
I know, it's hard to find sales on healthy frozen vegetables or meat, but when you do find them, buy as

much as you can afford. The good news is that since most of the approved items are either vegetable or meat, you can skip all of the rest of the aisles and concentrate all your efforts finding deals on produce, frozen veggies and meat.

Do the best you can.
There were many days when my budget dictated a "meat fast." I just couldn't pay the high price for a small piece of "approved meat" so I just didn't eat any. However, I don't expect that everyone wants to do the same thing, so if you can't afford grass fed beef, simply don't buy it, find a more affordable healthy substitute. Try ground pastured turkey. If that means you have to eat pastured chicken instead, then do that. There were many days when I found a can of wild caught tuna fish in olive oil could sustain me for a $1.50, so that was my meat for the day. If you can't manage the prices of pastured poultry, then shoot for as organic and healthy as you can. You're human, do your best.

Clothes
I was excited about achieving improved health and weight loss, but I hadn't account for the fact that I would need new clothes in progressively smaller sizes. I'm a teacher, so I buy the majority of my clothes at the beginning of the school year. I wish I had only bought a few things then and waited to buy more fitting clothing later.

It was exciting enough that I was buying a smaller size, but I didn't realize as the months passed that my clothes and underclothes would become unsightly lose. I don't think I've ever had the problem of my clothes being too big before. It was a good problem to have, but bad for my budget.

My advice to you about shopping for clothing:

Don't go on a big shopping spree.
After you reach your six-week mark or you have settled in the maintenance phase, buy your clothes in increments - a few at a time.

Wait for the sale.
You will be tempted to drape your new beautiful body in the most expensive of materials, but I assure you, if you spend too much money on expensive clothes, you will be mad when it no longer fits properly. However, expensive clothes do go on sale, you just have to wait for it. Your feelings won't be as hurt when it's time to retire it.

Once you reach your weight loss goals, if you can afford it, go ahead and splurge. Until then, I'll repeat: "Wait for the sale!"

Buy stretchy materials that can shrink with you.
Stretchy materials have saved my life - or at least kept me from going naked. If you buy stretchy clothes that

are a little snug at first, you'll get more wear out of them before they become too big.

Time constraints

Life gets busy. Who has time to cook every day? Not me! But the truth is, eating healthy food does take time, but not as much as we tend to think. There are ways to save time that make eating healthy manageable.

Steam veggies

It takes about 5-7 minutes to steam frozen broccoli/cauliflower. Coat with ghee (clarified butter) and salt and serve.

Raw veggies take no time to cook… literally

You don't have to cook most of the approved fresh veggies, so why not just eat them raw? Throw some fresh broccoli, cauliflower, or carrots in a bag and munch on them when you need a crunchy snack.

Tips for preparing meat

Baking requires less attention. So you can multi-task, if needed. Just place the meat on a pan, season and stick in the oven. Come back an hour later. But what if you don't have an hour? Pan searing or pan frying in an approved oil takes 10-15 minutes. You could also use an indoor grill such as a Foreman type and grill your meat in about 10 minutes, also. Or you can try my new favorite kitchen appliance: a pressure cooker. Pressure cookers such as "Insta-pot" cook foods quickly with high pressure. That means you can cook a roast in a portion of the time. I once pressured cooked a pork roast - from package to table in about 30 minutes. My husband watched skeptically as I prepared dinner. He was still doubtful, until he tasted that tender, succulent pulled pork.

So here's another reason to invest in a pressure cooker even if you don't plan to use it to cook beans or other "eat with caution" foods.

Cook large batches and freeze for later

I do most of my major cooking on my days off. I bake enough breakfast muffins to last throughout the week. Then I bake or fry enough meat to last a few days a time. Yes, that means most of the time you will be eating leftovers, but if you're busy like me, leftovers become lifesavers when you're time crunched.

Skin, skin... extra skin?

I had heard of people losing hundreds of pounds worth of weight only to be disappointed with their bodies because of extra skin. I heard of people paying thousands of dollars to get surgery for extreme cases of hanging skin. It doesn't matter how many times you here this happening to other people, nothing can prepare you for when it happens to you! That's why I'm here - to prepare you and to encourage you not to panic. It may seem so far away from now that the day will come when you will have lost so much weight and achieved your health goals and that the next obstacle will be your very own extra skin! But don't fret and don't rush to go get extra skin cut off unless it begins to cause a medical issue.

The biggest issue with extra skin is not a medical issue. It's usually a self-critical issue – we just don't like the way it looks. We lose the weight and yet, we still don't like what we see because things aren't hanging the way we expected. At that point, it's time to be less critical of that and more celebratory about the fact that you have lost weight and gained better health.

Before you consider getting surgery to fix your skin, it's better to instead, prepare your mind ahead of time so you'll know how to handle it. Don't end up despising your weight loss because of extra skin.

Here are some strategies for dealing with it:

Minimize the effect by losing weight slowly. Many of us are so excited about being a smaller size that we want to rush the process. Aside from being unhealthy, rapid weight loss can make it difficult for your skin to keep up. Just think, your body has been used to producing a certain amount of skins cells to cover your body, now all of a sudden, you don't need it. There's nowhere for it go and gravity is certainly going to have its way with every jiggly inch of it. So if no other reason, regulate your weight loss and take it slow. It's true that this new way of eating actually makes it easy to lose weight quickly, but do your best to lose no more than 10 pounds a month.

Tone it up

To combat the unsightly visual effects of extra skin, you should begin toning your muscles to offset this. After you've entered the 2-6 week phase and you feel comfortable with your new eating habits, you should begin working out with weights. No, you don't have to spend hours at the gym; you could spend as little as five minutes a day and still see results. I target multiple zones with each rep - I work both my arms and my legs simultaneously to save time. Search YouTube for programs that do the same. Look for five or 10 minute toning videos and use them to help you tone up.

Now, of course, if you've never trained with weights before, you should begin with light weights. Start with one pound weights and then work your way up to two, three, and up. Instead of being distracted by extra skin, you'll begin to notice better muscle tone and you'll be stronger, too!

Be patient

As I mentioned earlier, it took your body years to adjust to producing enough skin cells to cover your body. It's going to take just as much time or more to adjust to making less skin cells. If you were overweight X amount of years, you're going to have to be less weight for the same, if not more for your skin cells to get the message. Like I said, if your skin isn't causing you problems, give it time.

Recipes

Let me just say this: *you might get tired of eating the same thing over and over again.* So, figure out how you will spice things up ahead of time.

Get the *Plant Paradox Cookbook* or subscribe to Dr. Gundry's website: https://gundrymd.com/blog/
or YouTube channel:
https://www.youtube.com/channel/UCtxo0nTZjzlKJq5-vJq6s6g.

He posts regular cooking videos and recipes that are easy to make.

Another book that I've found helpful in discovering delicious, yet healthy recipes is Shelley Alexander's *Deliciously Holistic*. Some of the recipes contain ingredient that are on the "DO NOT EAT" list, so you may need to substitute them with something else or just leave them out completely. In addition to recipes, the book provides a useful list of healthy oils, along with their smoke point - which is important, so you'll know which oils you can use to cook or fry at high temperatures and which to use only as dressings. In this text, you'll also find an easy recipe for Ghee (clarified butter) and countless delicious smoothies.

The following are some recipes I've adapted to suit my own taste. They have are all Gundry-approved and husband-approved (if it can satisfy his keen chef's palate, I assure you, it will satisfy yours, too).

Blueberry Muffins

Makes about a dozen muffins

1 cup of coconut flour
1 cup of almond flour
1 cup of blueberries
⅔ cup of Extra Virgin Olive Oil
⅔ cup of Unrefined Coconut Oil
⅔ cup of water
6-7 eggs
5 teaspoons of baking powder
15-20 stevia packets
2 teaspoons of vanilla extract
1 teaspoon of cinnamon

Instructions:
Preheat the oven to 350 degrees.

Place all of the dry ingredients in a bowl and mix well: coconut flour, almond flour, baking powder, stevia, and cinnamon.

Next, add the olive oil and coconut oil into the dry ingredients. Stir in the vanilla extract, eggs and water. Use a hand or stand mixer to mix for approximately 1-2 minutes on medium to high.

Fold in the blueberries by hand.

Line a cupcake pan with paper liners. Fill each cup to the rim. Bake for approximately 15-20 minutes or until the tops are golden brown. Let the muffins cool for 5-10 minutes. You can eat them while they are still warm or freeze for later. (You can quickly thaw them by microwaving for 30-60 seconds)

Mint Chocolate Candy
Makes about 2 dozen pieces

1 package of 100% unsweetened chocolate (cacao)
1 cup of organic heavy whipping cream
½ cup of almonds
1 teaspoon of mint extract
10-15 packets of stevia (or sweeten to taste)

Instructions:
Pour the heavy whipping cream into a bowl. Add the chocolate. Slowly heat the mixture in 10-15 second intervals in the microwave. Whisk together until well mixed. Add mint extract. Stir in enough stevia until your desired level of sweetness has been reached. Fold in the almonds.

Spoon the mixture into small baking cups. Place in the freezer to harden the mixture for approximately 20 minutes. Store left over candy in the refrigerator.

Dark Chocolate Brownies

1 cup of coconut flour
1 cup of almond flour
½ cup of 100% unsweetened cocoa powder
⅔ cup of Extra Virgin Olive Oil
⅔ cup of Unrefined Coconut Oil
1 cup of water
6-7 eggs
5 teaspoons of baking powder
20-30 stevia packets
2 teaspoons of vanilla extract

Instructions:
Preheat the oven to 350 degrees.

Place all of the dry ingredients in a bowl and mix well: coconut flour, almond flour, cocoa powder, baking powder, and stevia.

Next, add the olive oil and coconut oil into the dry ingredients. Stir in the vanilla extract, eggs and water. Use a hand or stand mixer to mix for approximately 1-2 minutes on medium to high.

Pour the mixture into an oiled glass baking pan. Bake for approximately 15-20 minutes or until you can poke with a toothpick that comes out clean. Let the brownies cool for 5-10 minutes before cutting into squares.

Optional: Top with whipped cream (see next recipe). Use chocolate flavored whipped cream for added decadence.

Whipped Cream

1 cup of organic heavy whipping cream
4-5 packets of stevia (or sweeten to taste)

Optional:
1 teaspoon 100% unsweetened cocoa powder
½ teaspoon of vanilla extract (or other flavorings)

Instructions:
Mix the whipping cream and stevia in a bowl. (Add in optional ingredients to create different flavored whipped creams). Use a hand or stand mixer to mix on high for approximately 2-3 minutes. Whip until the mixture becomes light and fluffy. Store whipped cream in the refrigerator for up to a week.

Sweet Potato Fries

2-3 large organic sweet potatoes
Salt to taste
Avocado oil (or other approved oil that can withstand high cooking temperatures)

Instructions:
Preheat the oil on med/high heat.

Peel the potatoes (or leave skin on, if desired). Cut and slice into wedges or your desired thinness.

Carefully add fries to hot oil. Cook for approximately 10-15 minutes or until crisp and lightly browned. Remove from oil and place on a brown paper bag or paper towel to drain excess oil. Add salt to taste.

Baked Rosemary Salmon

4 oz. Salmon (fresh or frozen)
Sprig of Fresh Rosemary
1 tablespoon of Ghee or Extra Virgin Olive Oil
Salt & Pepper to taste

Instructions:
Preheat the oven to 350 degrees.

Grease the pan, and then coat the top of the salmon with ghee or olive oil. Chop rosemary leaves then sprinkle on top of salmon. Sprinkle with salt and pepper. Place in the oven for approximately 20 minutes or until meat springs back when touched.

Serve on a bed of lettuce or with steamed broccoli.

CHAPTER 7
GET HELP

Making life-changing choices about your health can be overwhelming. Sometimes, there's just one small detail that can make the all the difference between failure and success. Sometimes, all we need is someone who's been where we've been to coach us along.

I realize that different people have different levels of patience when it comes to reading and interpreting the details of Dr. Gundry's book. Some people I recommended it to, took it and were able to apply the concepts to their lives while others were overwhelmed by all of the information. As a teacher, I'm sensitive to this and understand that sometimes, you just need someone to tell you the most important points in simple, easy to digest terms. I've tried to do this with this book, but I realize some of you may still need more help.

For that reason, my mission is to help as many people as I can to achieve their health and wellness goals. Everyone, including you, deserves to feel energized; be healthy and happy. If I can do it, anyone can. It's as simple as that.

After reading this book, if you've made the choice to change your health, but you want some one-on-one guidance on how to integrate all these new habits into your life, I'd be happy to help you with a personalized 6-week coaching session.

6-Week Coaching Session Slots Available (Limited Time Only)

If you're ready to fully commit to changing your health and you need help establishing a new lifestyle, I can guide you through the process.

If you're interested in having me coach you through your weight-loss journey, just fill out an application at the following link:

Application:
https://goo.gl/forms/07jh9pTYPM7i81zK2

I will get in contact with you and schedule a time to talk with you to see how I can best help you. Together we will work to develop a plan to ensure your success.

I'm still a teacher, so I only have a **limited amount of coaching slots available** and will only coach for a limited time. So, if you think you might be interested, don't wait - slots for this limited time may fill up fast.

Got Questions? Comments?

I'm willing to help you however I can, so if you've got questions, or if you want to share your experiences or tell me about your success after trying this plan, please contact me at:

kiesha@kieshaeasley.com

I will get back to you within 24-48 hours.

You can also visit my website: www.kieshaeasley.com for more information. I'll be updating the site frequently with tips, recipes and other helpful information.

Join my email list to be the first to receive discounts, tips and updates: http://eepurl.com/dwgx3z

Thanks for reading! I wish you all the best as you set out on this journey to improve your health and increase your energy.

ABOUT
THE AUTHOR

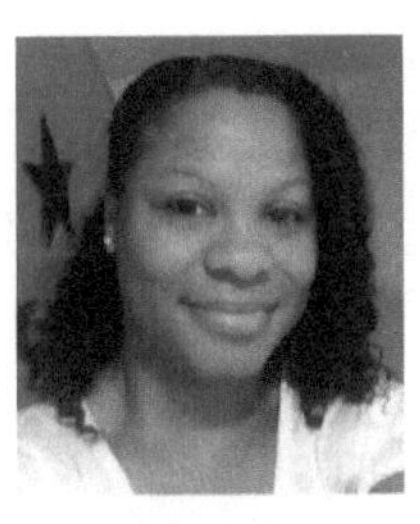

Kiesha R. Easley is a High School English Teacher, who got fed up with not having enough energy and mental strength to make it through the day. She knew that something had to give if she was going to continue working in such a fast-paced environment and keep up with her students.

She found a solution that transformed her life. In 2017, she started her journey and nearly a year later, she is 70 pounds lighter, looks 20 years younger and has more energy than ever before. She has regained her energy and health and wants to spread this message of healing.

Kiesha and her husband raise chickens, honeybees and a host of fruit trees in their backyard. Every year they plant a garden and grow many healthy leafy greens, herbs, and sweet potatoes. They grow and raise everything using only natural methods - no chemicals, pesticides or herbicides. So they benefit from the full health of the raw honey, fresh eggs, and vegetables that they harvest.

Email: kiesha@kieshaeasley.com
Website: www.kieshaeasley.com
Facebook: https://www.facebook.com/worthweight/
Twitter: https://twitter.com/kieshareasley

REFERENCES:
FOR FURTHER RESEARCH

7 Deadly Disruptors - Healthy substances that actually harm you. (2017, June 07). Retrieved from https://gundrymd.com/deadly-disruptors-plant-paradox/

Alexander, S. (2013). *Deliciously holistic cookbook: Healing foods, recipes and lifestyle tips to help increase your energy and immunity.* Loa Angeles, CA: Harmony Publishing.

B Vitamins. (2018, March 06). Retrieved from https://medlineplus.gov/bvitamins.html

Gundry, S. R., & Buehl, O. B. (2017). *The plant paradox: The hidden dangers in "healthy" foods that cause disease and weight gain.* New York: Harper Wave.

Omega-3 fats: Good for your heart: MedlinePlus Medical Encyclopedia. (n.d.). Retrieved from https://medlineplus.gov/ency/patientinstructions/000767.htm

The Plant Paradox Approved Foods (print-friendly list). (2018, May 02). Retrieved from https://gundrymd.com/plant-paradox-shopping-list/

Turner, C. W. (2008). *My seven-day makeover: One breast cancer survivor's spiritual journey.* Champaign, IL: 4044 Pub.

Understand Your Risk for Excessive Blood Clotting. (n.d.). Retrieved from http://www.heart.org/HEARTORG/Conditions/More/Understand-Your-Risk-for-Excessive-Blood-Clotting_UCM_448771_Article.jsp#.WxXttyAh1UQ

Vitamin D. (2018, April 16). Retrieved from https://medlineplus.gov/vitamind.html

W. (n.d.). What Are Ketones? Retrieved from
        https://www.perfectketo.com/what-are-
        ketones/

INDEX: